Just Br

21 day breathing exercise plan for asthma

Based on the system developed in Russia by Dr K P Buteyko (1923 – 2003)

by J L Brindley

First Published in the UK 2003
Revised Edition 2005

Published and distributed by J L Brindley

ISBN: 0-9551488-0-4 (10 digit) 978-0-9551488-0-4 (13 digit)

IMPORTANT CAUTIONS

Please note the following cautions before using the booklet.

To reduce the risk of injury, never force or strain during exercises. If you experience pain or discomfort, stop immediately and consult your doctor.

Other special cautions may apply to individuals with specific health issues. For that reason, you should consult your doctor to find out if special restrictions apply to you. For that reason, this book is sold without any warranties or guarantees of any kind.

Any liability, loss or damage in connection with any use of this booklet including but not limited to any liability, loss or damage resulting from the performance of the exercises or the advice and information given here, is expressly disclaimed.

1 - Introduction

Asthma can quickly take your breath away!

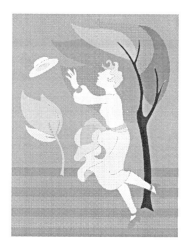

But something as simple as changing your breathing can make a world of difference.

The exact cause of asthma is not known. It is likely that many factors are involved such as the genes inherited from parents, antibiotic use, central heating, more families having cats and dogs and perhaps the lower temperatures we now use to wash clothes and bedding.

There is no cure for asthma. The majority of asthmatics are treated with inhalers and medicines designed to suppress symptoms.

Breathing exercises provide another option, an option which offers you safe and effective techniques to help you to reduce and manage symptoms.

By following this programme you will begin to understand how asthma and breathing are related. This leads to a new confidence in controlling asthma and most people find that they are able to reduce their medication and start feeling better and better.

Just Breathe is a 21-day breathing exercise plan designed to restore your natural breathing pattern.

How to use this book

Regular practice

Our breathing style has developed over many years and is as much a part of us as the way we walk. Improving our breathing means going back to basics and restoring our normal healthy rhythm.

Imagine our breathing pattern is set by a sophisticated clock in the brain. The exercises help to reset this internal breathing clock to the correct time.

It is rather like learning to ride a bike. You can talk about it, think about it or write about it but the only way to be successful is to practise!

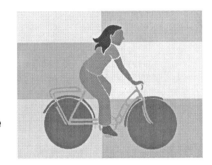

Correcting bad breathing will not happen overnight, but by following the programme most people see positive results after just one week.

One step at a time

Work through each section before moving on.

Most of the breathing exercises appear simple and easy. You may think a section doesn't apply and be tempted to jump ahead or rush through to the end. Don't!

Try to keep to the programme as the first stage, **Set A,** establishes important elements such as posture and relaxation : making the second stage, **Set B,** easier to master.

2 – Getting Started

Be vigilant! Only nose-breathe

Think about it - the nose is for designed for breathing and the mouth for eating.

Your first challenge in this breathing improvement programme is to only use your nose for breathing – both in and out – all the time.

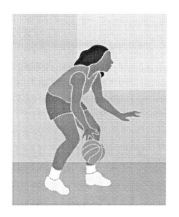

The nose isn't just the part you see, there is a big area behind it, which acts as a super-efficient air-cleaning machine.

Breathing through the nose prevents pollen, dust and other small particles from entering the lungs. These can irritate the sensitive lining of the lungs causing breathlessness, wheezing and coughing. The nose also warms and moistens the air and makes a gas that helps to keep the lungs healthy.

Check whether you are nose-breathing now. Asthmatics often breathe through their mouth and all the benefits of nose-breathing are lost. From this day on, try to never mouth-breathe again!

Ask friends and family to help by letting you know if you are breathing through your mouth.

To really make your nose start working properly you will need to practise the **Nose-Clearing Exercises** (shown on the next page) at least twice every day for the next three weeks.

Nose-Clearing Exercises

Remember to breathe normally (not deeply) throughout, and only through the nose.

---

1. Move the head backwards and forwards very slowly.
Notice how heavy your head is.
Feel the weight of the head for a moment as you go back and for a moment as the head drops forward.
Repeat six times.

2. Breathe in as you move the head slowly backwards and breathe out as you move the head slowly forwards.
Breathe normally but slowly.
Repeat six times.

3. After a normal breath out, hold your nose.
Nod your head backwards and forwards three times.
Let go and breathe in and out slowly through your nose.
Repeat three times.

4. After a normal breath out, hold your nose.
Blow gently but don't let any air escape.
This is the same feeling as clearing your ears in the swimming pool.
Repeat six times.

Practise nose-clearing at least twice a day, but if your nose keeps blocking or you have rhinitis, you can repeat the exercises up to six times daily.

Caution : Seek medical advice before practising these exercises
if you have an **ear, nose or throat infection**

Techniques

Let your breathing relax

Try to sense your normal breathing for a couple of minutes. Put one hand on your upper chest and the other below your ribs, just above your navel.

If you can allow your breathing to relax, only the lower hand will move. Many asthmatics unconsciously breathe using mainly the upper chest muscles. Sitting comfortably upright helps you to relax and breathe correctly.

Pulse
You may wish to check your wrist pulse as a measure of relaxation.

A Control Pause (CP)
After a normal breath **out** pinch your nose.

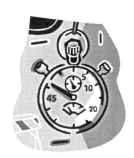

Let go at the first sign of discomfort and breathe in quietly through your nose. Note the time in seconds that you were able to hold your breath. After 'letting go', you should be able to breathe through your nose as normal and not need to gasp.

Slow Breathing

Look at the second hand of a clock or watch and allow your breathing to become slower **without making it deeper.**

Try breathing in for three seconds, out for three seconds and holding for one second - **3 : 3 : 1 rhythm** for one to two minutes.

Once this is comfortable you can gradually slow your breathing even more. Breathing in for four seconds, out for five seconds, holding for one second - **4 : 5 : 1 rhythm** for one to two minutes.

Starting to practise

The techniques on the previous page are brought together in a exercise session called **Set A**. Combining **Slow Breathing** with gentle **Control Pauses** may seem tedious but establishes important elements such as getting into a regular focused routine, and allowing your breathing to settle into a comfortable pattern.

Ideally, sets should be practised before breakfast, lunch and sleep. It is preferable not to practise immediately after meals.

Relaxation

As Lao Tzu said in 500 B.C. "The perfect man breathes as if he is not breathing." The key to doing this is the ability to relax which many people cannot easily achieve.

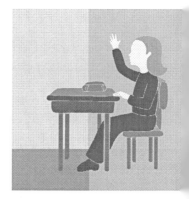

To help yourself relax you can use cushions to support your back and it is a good idea to plant your feet on the floor.

Air hunger

During the breathing sets you should feel a slight breathlessness or shortage of air which is called "air hunger".

Just a hint of air hunger is a good thing but too much will make you feel tense and stressed. By trying too hard, the practice can become ineffective because the relaxation element is lost.

By immediately following the Control Pause with slow, relaxed breathing you should maintain a small feeling of beneficial air hunger throughout.

Air hunger is an essential part of the exercise.

Set A

Pulse then *Control Pause*
⇩
Immediately followed by
3 minutes Slow Breathing
⇩

Rest *for 15 to 30 seconds*
⇩

Control Pause
⇩
3 minutes Slow Breathing
⇩

Rest *for 15 to 30 seconds*
⇩

Control Pause
⇩
3 minutes of Slow breathing
⇩

Rest *for 15 to 30 seconds*
⇩

Control Pause
⇩
3 minutes Slow Breathing

Rest *for 30 seconds*

⇩
Final Control Pause and *Pulse*

3 - Asthma Management

Asthma medication

Even if you feel much better you must continue to take your asthma medication until you have spoken to your doctor.

At the first signs of breathlessness, you might like to try the slow breathing exercise for three minutes. Sometimes this can stop the symptoms but ensure you continue to carry your reliever with you and use it when needed.

Nose-breathe all the time

Establishing a nose-breathing habit can be difficult. Sometimes as soon as your mind is elsewhere your mouth automatically opens!

Using paper- tape can help reinforce the new habit. Coat the lips with lipsalve and put a small piece of paper-tape across your mouth to encourage nose-breathing. By doing this while you are sitting watching TV or reading a book you will naturally be practising a breathing exercise.

Daily walk

Include a fifteen minute nose-breathing walk in your daily programme (no talking allowed!)

Week 1 Chart

Day	Nose-Clearing morning	Set A Morning Final CP	Daily walk	Set A afternoon Final CP	Paper-tape for one hour	Nose-Clearing evening	Set A evening Final CP
1							
2							
3							
4							
5							
6							
7							

Key elements of practice:
Nose-breathing
Quiet breathing
Relaxed breathing
Lower-chest breathing
Your pulse should be less at the end of the Set

Your Control Pause should gradually increase during the week.

4 – Everyday Situations

Sudden symptoms

Asthma attacks can sometimes begin with little warning. Often exposure to an allergen such as cat hair or an irritant like cigarette smoke can be the cause. Sometimes though, the attack can be the result of a change in breathing style.

As an example, many asthmatics find that when they are enjoying themselves and laughing out loud they become breathless and need a puff of their inhaler. Similarly, asthma symptoms can start after walking uphill, coughing or even talking on the telephone.

All these situations can cause people with asthma to breathe too much. You breathe like an elephant and you need to breathe like a mouse! The Quick Fix technique can help to stop 'over-breathing'.

 Quick Fix

After a **normal breath out**, hold your breath for 10 counts.
⇩

Take 20 **very small, silent** breaths through the nose.
⇩

Breathe in and out normally through the nose.

You can repeat the Quick Fix two or three times
But if you still feel breathless **use your blue reliever inhaler** as usual.

Coughing

For many people coughing can start or
worsen asthma symptoms.

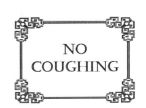

Where the cough is dry and tickly the
simplest and best advice is - don't cough.

The more you cough the more you will feel
like coughing!

At first it will be difficult to overcome the desire to cough. For many
years you may have been coughing just to "get it over with" or
because it happens automatically.

A dry cough is a type of irritation that can be caused by several
factors such as cold, dry or fast-moving air hitting the throat.

Once you have coughed, you will normally feel the need to take a
big breath and cough again. You are effectively 'feeding' the cough
as each big breath further irritates the lungs and throat.

The **anti-coughing exercise** is
designed to help reduce an
over-sensitive cough reflex.

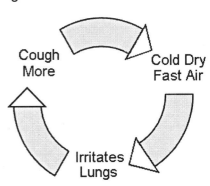

If you can reduce the air flow and
keep the air around the throat warm
and moist it is often possible to stop a
cough at an early stage.

To gain most benefit the exercise should be practised to counteract
a "pretend" cough several times a day.

Anti-Coughing Exercise

At the first tickling feeling of cough
⇩

Put your hand over your mouth.

Swallow

Keep your hand over your mouth throughout
⇩

Take a small breath in and out, pinch your nose

Hold your breath for five to ten counts
⇩

Release the nose but leave the hand over the mouth
⇩

Breathe **small, careful breaths** through the nose for 30 seconds

All the time resisting the urge to cough
⇩

Take a slow, steady breath in and out of the nose
⇩

Repeat the practice twice more
or
until the 'tickle' has subsided.

If you have a **productive cough** and are coughing anything other than small
amounts of clear mucus, you will need to see your doctor
as you may have a chest infection or another condition.

5 – Increasing Air Hunger

During the second and third weeks, the focus is on breathing less and less. Using new techniques and building on the first week of training we seek to reduce breathing volume further. The aim is to become accustomed to a feeling of "air hunger" lasting several minutes.

As with any skill, practice is essential for success.
During Weeks 2 and 3, the nose-clearing exercises and Set should be practised three times a day.

Extended Pause [Optional Technique]

After a normal breath out, pinch your nose
⇩

Instead of releasing after the comfortable control pause time
Extend the breath-hold by an extra 5 seconds
⇩
Release and control your breathing

You must be able to breathe in through your nose when you stop.

Practising an Extended Pause can be easier if you use 'distraction' techniques such as walking or stretching. Do not gulp air.

Warning: Do not practise Extended Pause if you have
high blood pressure, a heart condition, epilepsy, diabetes
or any other severe health problem.

Reduced Breathing

Reduced (Volume) Breathing focuses on breathing less air without strict timing. You maintain a gentle flow of air but with slightly smaller breaths than normal.

Bring one hand just above the navel
Establish normal relaxed breathing
⇩

Make each breath a little smaller
Relax
Settle into this pattern for about 30 seconds
⇩

Introduce a pause between the small breaths
Follow the pattern in …out… pause
⇩

Once settled in this pattern increase the length of the pause without increasing the size of each breath.

Sit comfortably and regularly check for tension

Gradually you will find you are hardly breathing but feel quite comfortable and peaceful

---

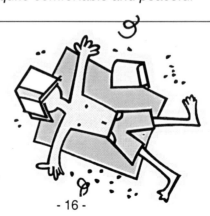

Set B

Set B combines all the techniques covered so far into a
15 - 20 minute breathing exercise.

Pulse and Starting Control Pause (CP)
⇩
Slow Breathing 3 minutes
⇩
Rest for 15 to 30 seconds

Extended Pause
⇩
Reduced Breathing 3 minutes
⇩
Rest for 15 to 30 seconds

Control Pause
⇩
Reduced Breathing 3 minutes
⇩
Rest for 15 to 30 seconds

Extended Pause
⇩
Reduced Breathing 3 minutes
⇩
Rest for 30 seconds

Final Control Pause(CP) and Pulse

Your Final CP should be higher than your Starting CP.

6 – Asthma Tips

Breathing at Night

Nose-breathing is so important that it helps if you can breathe through your nose even while asleep. A simple way to achieve this is by taping your lips at night. Just before sleeping:

1. Coat the lips with lip salve
2. Tear off a small piece of paper-tape
3. Turn over the ends
4. Stick vertically over mouth

This technique holds the lips together whilst allowing you to breathe through the sides of your mouth if necessary.

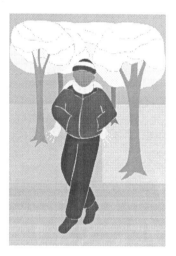

Avoiding Colds

Colds can make asthma worse for a short time.

Frequently washing your hands can help you to avoid catching colds and flu.

The main way you get a cold is not from people sneezing in your face but by picking up the virus on your own hands.

Week 2 Chart

Day	Nose-Clearing morning	Set B Morning Final CP	Daily walk	Set B Afternoon Final CP	Nose-Clearing evening	Set B Evening Final CP	Tape at Night
8							
9							
10							
11							
12							
13							
14							

Week 3 Chart

Day	Nose-Clearing morning	Set B Morning Final CP	Daily walk	Set B Afternoon Final CP	Nose-Clearing evening	Set B Evening Final CP	Tape at Night
15							
16							
17							
18							
19							
20							
21							

Frequently Asked Questions

Do I have to pinch my nose?
No, you can just hold your breath, but holding your nose is more effective.

When should I stop my Control Pause?
Start with a short pause of say 3 seconds, at the end of which you should definitely not experience lack of air. Repeat the pause adding 2 seconds each time. When you finally feel a slight lack of air, this is your control pause.

Have I got a cold?
Many asthmatics find at the end of the first week they have cold-like symptoms: a runny nose for example. This is a good sign as it indicates your nose is becoming clear. The symptoms usually disappear after a few more days.

What do I do after 21 days?
If you have found the exercises helpful you may wish to continue until your control pause is over 30. Then you can begin to build the principles into your life and gradually cut down the number of sets you practise.

What if I practise but my control pause has not increased?
You may be making a simple error and need to see a breathing teacher.

What if I start panicking when I do reduced breathing?
You are probably associating reduced breathing with an asthma attack. Use only slow breathing.

What do I do if I feel chest pain when I practise the exercises?
If you regularly feel chest pain you should consult your doctor. Otherwise, you might be controlling your breathing by tensing your chest muscles. Focus on relaxing your shoulders and back.

My asthma is getting worse even though I am practising ?
Consult your doctor; you may have a problem unrelated to the exercises or you are practising incorrectly. You may need to see a breathing teacher

Who devised these exercises?
They are based on the breathing approach developed by the Ukrainian, Dr Konstantin Buteyko and on therapeutic yoga practices.

A Severe Asthma Attack

We all hope that it doesn't happen, but sometimes asthmatics can experience severe attacks. These may occur quickly or build up over days or weeks. It is important to recognise the severity of the situation.

Often it is obvious that an attack is becoming out of control when the asthmatic is wheezing or appears distressed. However, even during a severe attack some asthmatics may not appear distressed, which can make recognition of the warning signs difficult for other people.

> Seek immediate medical assistance if an asthma sufferer shows **ANY** of the following symptoms:

Cannot complete sentences
Blue around the lips and face
Tired and struggling to breathe
Has a breathing rate more than about 30 breaths each minute
Blue reliever inhaler seems ineffective
Peak Flow less than 50% of best ever reading

The exercises in this book are not helpful for anyone who is experiencing a severe asthma attack.

If in doubt do not hesitate to contact your doctor,

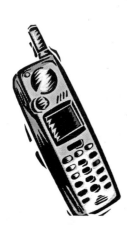

or **Asthma UK adviceline**

08457 01 02 03, Monday-Friday, 9am-5pm

or **NHS Direct 0845-46-47**

NHS Direct is a 24 hour confidential helpline providing advice and information on what to do about health concerns.

7 - Further Information

Janet Brindley Registered Buteyko teacher., B.Sc(Hons)., BWY Dip.
Janet started her career as a medical researcher and hospital scientist. As a life long asthmatic, she has personally experienced the benefits of breathing exercises.

Janet teaches the *Just Breathe 21 day exercise plan* at the Brentwood Clinic, 31, Shenfield Road, Brentwood, Essex CM15 8AG.

If you would like an appointment

please telephone　　 01277 364 724

or email info@breathingteacher.co.uk
www.breathingteacher.co.uk

Buteyko Breathing Association

The Buteyko Breathing Association is a non-profit making organisation committed to improving the health of asthmatics and those with breathing-related problems.

Buteyko Breathing Association teachers are health professionals who have been trained to teach Dr Buteyko's breathing exercises.

Ring the 24 hour ansaphone line　 01277 366 906
for a list of registered Buteyko teachers.

Asthma UK

Asthma UK is the charity dedicated to improving the health and well-being of the 5.2 million people in the UK whose lives are affected by asthma.

08457 01 02 03

Practising Buteyko CD

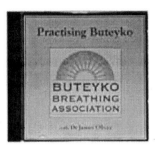

Dr James Oliver is a General Practitioner based in Cornwall.

You may find this CD helpful if you are practising the breathing exercises using this book

Track List

Buteyko basics

1. Introduction
2. Breath Following
3. Control Pause
4. Extended Pause
5. Slow Breathing
6. Reduced Volume Breathing

Buteyko Practice

7. Nose Clearing exercises
8. Buteyko Exercise Set A (as page 9)
9. Buteyko Exercise Set B (as page 17)

This CD is available from The Buteyko Shop online at

www.thebuteykoshop.co.uk

or by post - see details on the back cover

Please note: Dr Oliver has produced this CD primarily to assist students who are working with a Registered Buteyko teacher.